MW01533827

ONE DAY AT A TIME

Daily Affirmations and Encouragement
for the Breastfeeding Mother

ONE DAY AT A TIME

by Keleigh Crigler Hadley

Copyright 2011 by Keleigh Crigler Hadley

Cover Photograph by Kristopher Crigler

All rights reserved.

No portion of this book may be reproduced-mechanically, electronically, or by any other means, including photocopying-without written permission of the author.

ISBN:978-1456538507

Note: All children are unique and this book is not intended to substitute for the advice of your pediatrician or other physician who should be consulted on infant matters, especially when a baby shows signs of illness or unusual behavior. Please note, I do realize breastfeeding is not for everyone. I also want you to know that you are in no way a failure if you decide that breastfeeding just isn't for you.

Also by Keleigh Crigler Hadley

Preacher's Kids: Secrets & Salvation

Preacher's Kids: Wicked & Wise

This book is lovingly dedicated to my m&m's:

Malcolm Mckinsey Hadley -the light of my life.

McKenna Drew Hadley – my heart and joy.

This book is also dedicated to all mothers: especially my mom–
Ellen Crigler.

What is an affirmation? Affirmations are simple. They are you being in conscious control of your thoughts. Thinking, saying, or writing affirmations is an easy way to bring positive change into your life. Amazing results in life come when we change our habits. Our habits change when we have a change in attitude. Affirmations are a way we can change our attitudes.

Four days after my son Malcolm was born, he was hospitalized for severe jaundice. I wasn't able to nurse so I pumped. Unfortunately, I was never able to fully provide enough milk to breastfeed exclusively but I supplemented for eight months. I knew that even an ounce of 'liquid gold' was better than none at all.

When my daughter McKenna was born I was determined to nurse her. I prepared my body by taking herbal supplements and teas that promoted breastfeeding. I *prepared my mind* by reading positive affirmations about the benefits of breastfeeding daily.

Sow a thought and you reap an action; sow an act and you reap a habit; sow a habit and you reap a character; sow a character and you reap a destiny. --
Ralph Waldo Emerson

1

Do affirmations really work? YES!

The reason why affirmations work is because affirmations are the 'code', the 'language', the natural way your mind does business. Self-talk - the traffic of your brain - starts out as an affirmation from the outside. These affirmations are either created by you or given to you by others. They are the statements that you repeat to yourself on a daily basis.

My hope is that you will read the affirmations in this book on a daily basis and strengthen your resolve to provide your child with the <u>very best nutrition possible.</u>

DAY 1

I am giving my baby the *perfect* infant nutrition.

Doesn't it feel amazing to know that your baby is eating pure, clean, healthy breastmilk that was designed just for him/her?

_____

_____

_____

_____

_____

_____

_____

_____

Time	Minutes on breast		Diaper Changes	
	L	**R**	Pee	Poop
	L	**R**	Pee	Poop
	L	**R**	Pee	Poop
	L	**R**	Pee	Poop
	L	**R**	Pee	Poop
	L	**R**	Pee	Poop
	L	**R**	Pee	Poop
	L	**R**	Pee	Poop
	L	**R**	Pee	Poop
	L	**R**	Pee	Poop
	L	**R**	Pee	Poop
	L	**R**	Pee	Poop

DAY 2

Colostrum is a *superfood* for my baby.

There is so much talk in the media about superfoods – acai, blueberries, wheatgrass, etc. You have within you the ULTIMATE superfood! Colostrum provides not only perfect nutrition tailored to the needs of your newborn, but also large amounts of living cells which will defend your baby against many harmful agents. The concentration of immune factors is much higher in colostrum than in mature milk.

Colostrum actually works as a natural and 100% safe vaccine. It contains large quantities of an antibody called secretory immunoglobulin A (IgA)

Time	Minutes on breast		Diaper Changes	
	L	R	Pee	Poop
	L	R	Pee	Poop
	L	R	Pee	Poop
	L	R	Pee	Poop
	L	R	Pee	Poop
	L	R	Pee	Poop
	L	R	Pee	Poop
	L	R	Pee	Poop
	L	R	Pee	Poop
	L	R	Pee	Poop
	L	R	Pee	Poop
	L	R	Pee	Poop

7

I am *bonding* with my baby.

Scientists have discovered the secret behind how breastfeeding helps mothers bond with their babies. A study has revealed that the action of a baby suckling actually changes how the mother's brain behaves. This results in a massive rush of the 'love hormone' oxytocin in women's brains. The release of the chemical in massive surges enhances a mother's feelings of trust, love and affection, scientists say.

Time	Minutes on breast		Diaper Changes	
	L	**R**	Pee	Poop
	L	**R**	Pee	Poop
	L	**R**	Pee	Poop
	L	**R**	Pee	Poop
	L	**R**	Pee	Poop
	L	**R**	Pee	Poop
	L	**R**	Pee	Poop
	L	**R**	Pee	Poop
	L	**R**	Pee	Poop
	L	**R**	Pee	Poop
	L	**R**	Pee	Poop
	L	**R**	Pee	Poop

DAY 4

Breastfeeding my baby is developing healthy brain *growth*.

Studies have recently shown that breastfed infants have higher concentration levels of DHA in their brain tissue. DHA and other fats in the breast milk contribute directly to brain growth by providing the right substances for manufacturing myelin, the fatty sheath that surrounds nerve fibers, insulating them so that these pathways can carry information. Also, breast milk is rich in cholesterol; formula contains none. Cholesterol provides basic components for building the brain and manufacturing hormones and vitamin D. (Higher dietary cholesterol at the stage of fastest brain growth - what a smart idea!)

Time	Minutes on breast		Diaper Changes	
	L	R	Pee	Poop
	L	R	Pee	Poop
	L	R	Pee	Poop
	L	R	Pee	Poop
	L	R	Pee	Poop
	L	R	Pee	Poop
	L	R	Pee	Poop
	L	R	Pee	Poop
	L	R	Pee	Poop
	L	R	Pee	Poop
	L	R	Pee	Poop
	L	R	Pee	Poop

DAY 5

My breastmilk is *ideal* for my preemie.

The breastmilk of mothers who deliver prematurely is ideally suited to the special needs of the premature baby. Colostrum and breastmilk contain white blood cells, antibodies and other valuable immune properties that may help a premature baby resist infection. Recent studies have shown that breast milk may improve the neurological development of premature infants.

Time	Minutes on breast		Diaper Changes	
	L	R	Pee	Poop
	L	R	Pee	Poop
	L	R	Pee	Poop
	L	R	Pee	Poop
	L	R	Pee	Poop
	L	R	Pee	Poop
	L	R	Pee	Poop
	L	R	Pee	Poop
	L	R	Pee	Poop
	L	R	Pee	Poop
	L	R	Pee	Poop
	L	R	Pee	Poop

DAY 6

My breastmilk is *free.*

Everyone knows that babies are expensive. Breastfeeding can help you save **$1300-2000** per year in feeding costs. An additional $340- $450 per year is saved in doctor co-pay visits because breastfed babies get sick less often.

Time	Minutes on breast		Diaper Changes	
	L	**R**	Pee	Poop
	L	**R**	Pee	Poop
	L	**R**	Pee	Poop
	L	**R**	Pee	Poop
	L	**R**	Pee	Poop
	L	**R**	Pee	Poop
	L	**R**	Pee	Poop
	L	**R**	Pee	Poop
	L	**R**	Pee	Poop
	L	**R**	Pee	Poop
	L	**R**	Pee	Poop
	L	**R**	Pee	Poop

DAY 7

My breastmilk will help *prevent* infection.

Your breastfed child will not only have fewer ear infections, but protection against other infections. Breastfeeding provides protection against diarrhea, gastrointestinal and respiratory infections; in fact, infections of every kind.

Time	Minutes on breast		Diaper Changes	
	L	**R**	Pee	Poop
	L	**R**	Pee	Poop
	L	**R**	Pee	Poop
	L	**R**	Pee	Poop
	L	**R**	Pee	Poop
	L	**R**	Pee	Poop
	L	**R**	Pee	Poop
	L	**R**	Pee	Poop
	L	**R**	Pee	Poop
	L	**R**	Pee	Poop
	L	**R**	Pee	Poop
	L	**R**	Pee	Poop

17

DAY 8

My breastmilk will help my baby gain *healthy* weight.

Because premature babies usually weigh very little at birth, good growth is important for their development. Breast milk contains lipase, which helps premature babies digest the fats in breast milk more completely. Better fat absorption is an important benefit of breastfeeding a premature baby.

_____

_____

_____

_____

_____

_____

Time	Minutes on breast		Diaper Changes	
	L	**R**	Pee	Poop
	L	**R**	Pee	Poop
	L	**R**	Pee	Poop
	L	**R**	Pee	Poop
	L	**R**	Pee	Poop
	L	**R**	Pee	Poop
	L	**R**	Pee	Poop
	L	**R**	Pee	Poop
	L	**R**	Pee	Poop
	L	**R**	Pee	Poop
	L	**R**	Pee	Poop
	L	**R**	Pee	Poop

DAY 9

My breastmilk *adapts* to my baby needs.

Amazingly, your breastmilk adapts its composition from day to day to suit the changing needs of your baby.
Your baby's rapidly growing body needs these nutrients for the proper development of the brain, nerve tissues, and cell membranes.

Time	Minutes on breast		Diaper Changes	
	L	R	Pee	Poop
	L	R	Pee	Poop
	L	R	Pee	Poop
	L	R	Pee	Poop
	L	R	Pee	Poop
	L	R	Pee	Poop
	L	R	Pee	Poop
	L	R	Pee	Poop
	L	R	Pee	Poop
	L	R	Pee	Poop
	L	R	Pee	Poop
	L	R	Pee	Poop

21

DAY 10

My breastmilk helps to *prevent* colic.

The causes of colic are not completely known, but there is one thing we know for sure: a baby who is not completely satisfied with what she has eaten is going to be fussy. If baby never quite gets satisfied, she is going to be fussy for long periods of time. Whatever you do, don't get frustrated and give up breastfeeding. Bottle fed babies get colic, too. Some studies seem to indicate that they get it more frequently.

Time	Minutes on breast		Diaper Changes	
	L	**R**	Pee	Poop
	L	**R**	Pee	Poop
	L	**R**	Pee	Poop
	L	**R**	Pee	Poop
	L	**R**	Pee	Poop
	L	**R**	Pee	Poop
	L	**R**	Pee	Poop
	L	**R**	Pee	Poop
	L	**R**	Pee	Poop
	L	**R**	Pee	Poop
	L	**R**	Pee	Poop
	L	**R**	Pee	Poop

DAY 11

Breastfeeding makes me *feel* good!

Not only does breastfeeding benefit your body, it helps your mind, too. The same hormones that help make milk help a mother feel peaceful. When you sit down to breastfeed, you may find yourself drifting off to sleep. If you've been feeling stressed or harried, breastfeeding brings a sense of contentment and relaxation. This may be prolactin at work, since prolactin is known to be one of the body's stress-fighting hormones, and research has shown that breastfeeding mothers are more tolerant of stress.

Time	Minutes on breast		Diaper Changes	
	L	**R**	Pee	Poop
	L	**R**	Pee	Poop
	L	**R**	Pee	Poop
	L	**R**	Pee	Poop
	L	**R**	Pee	Poop
	L	**R**	Pee	Poop
	L	**R**	Pee	Poop
	L	**R**	Pee	Poop
	L	**R**	Pee	Poop
	L	**R**	Pee	Poop
	L	**R**	Pee	Poop
	L	**R**	Pee	Poop

DAY 12

Breastfeeding my *baby* helps prevent diaper rash.

Breast-fed babies have a lower incidence of diaper rash, possibly because their stools have higher pH and lower enzymatic activity .

Time	Minutes on breast		Diaper Changes	
	L	**R**	Pee	Poop
	L	**R**	Pee	Poop
	L	**R**	Pee	Poop
	L	**R**	Pee	Poop
	L	**R**	Pee	Poop
	L	**R**	Pee	Poop
	L	**R**	Pee	Poop
	L	**R**	Pee	Poop
	L	**R**	Pee	Poop
	L	**R**	Pee	Poop
	L	**R**	Pee	Poop
	L	**R**	Pee	Poop

27

DAY 13

Breastfeeding my baby means I don't have to *sterilize* bottles.

With everything that you have to do for your precious child, things could get a little hectic. Isn't it nice that there is one less thing you have to do?

Time	Minutes on breast		Diaper Changes	
	L	R	Pee	Poop
	L	R	Pee	Poop
	L	R	Pee	Poop
	L	R	Pee	Poop
	L	R	Pee	Poop
	L	R	Pee	Poop
	L	R	Pee	Poop
	L	R	Pee	Poop
	L	R	Pee	Poop
	L	R	Pee	Poop
	L	R	Pee	Poop
	L	R	Pee	Poop

Breastfeeding will help prevent

obesity in my baby

Breastfeeding longer than three months can cut a child's risk of later becoming overweight or obese by more than 40 percent!

Time	Minutes on breast		Diaper Changes	
	L	R	Pee	Poop
	L	R	Pee	Poop
	L	R	Pee	Poop
	L	R	Pee	Poop
	L	R	Pee	Poop
	L	R	Pee	Poop
	L	R	Pee	Poop
	L	R	Pee	Poop
	L	R	Pee	Poop
	L	R	Pee	Poop
	L	R	Pee	Poop
	L	R	Pee	Poop

31

Breastfeeding my baby is *healthier* for ME!

A new study published in *The American Journal of Medicine* suggests that women who breast-feed for at least one month have a decreased risk of breast and ovarian cancers and Type 2 Diabetes.

_____

_____

_____

_____

_____

_____

_____

_____

_____

_____

_____

_____

_____

_____

_____

_____

_____

Time	Minutes on breast		Diaper Changes	
	L	R	Pee	Poop
	L	R	Pee	Poop
	L	R	Pee	Poop
	L	R	Pee	Poop
	L	R	Pee	Poop
	L	R	Pee	Poop
	L	R	Pee	Poop
	L	R	Pee	Poop
	L	R	Pee	Poop
	L	R	Pee	Poop
	L	R	Pee	Poop
	L	R	Pee	Poop

DAY 16

Breastfeeding gives my baby *sweet* smelling breath and poop!

You can return that Diaper Genie for something more useful because there is no need to cover up odors when you breastfeed.

Time	Minutes on breast		Diaper Changes	
	L	**R**	Pee	Poop
	L	**R**	Pee	Poop
	L	**R**	Pee	Poop
	L	**R**	Pee	Poop
	L	**R**	Pee	Poop
	L	**R**	Pee	Poop
	L	**R**	Pee	Poop
	L	**R**	Pee	Poop
	L	**R**	Pee	Poop
	L	**R**	Pee	Poop
	L	**R**	Pee	Poop
	L	**R**	Pee	Poop

I am getting back to my pre-baby weight *faster*

Breastfeeding burns calories. Over 600 calories a day for breastfeeding women who don't supplement with formula. 600 calories! That's like getting two hours of aerobic exercise each day. A study published in the Journal of American Dietician Association shows breastfeeding melts off inches around your hips and butt.

Time	Minutes on breast		Diaper Changes	
	L	**R**	Pee	Poop
	L	**R**	Pee	Poop
	L	**R**	Pee	Poop
	L	**R**	Pee	Poop
	L	**R**	Pee	Poop
	L	**R**	Pee	Poop
	L	**R**	Pee	Poop
	L	**R**	Pee	Poop
	L	**R**	Pee	Poop
	L	**R**	Pee	Poop
	L	**R**	Pee	Poop
	L	**R**	Pee	Poop

DAY 18

Breastfeeding is sanitary and my milk is always the *perfect* temperature.

Every year babies are burned from drinking milk from a bottle that is too hot. Bottle fed babies also have a higher number of stomach illnesses from improperly cleaned bottles or milk that has spoiled.

_____

_____

_____

_____

_____

_____

_____

_____

_____

_____

Time	Minutes on breast		Diaper Changes	
	L	R	Pee	Poop
	L	R	Pee	Poop
	L	R	Pee	Poop
	L	R	Pee	Poop
	L	R	Pee	Poop
	L	R	Pee	Poop
	L	R	Pee	Poop
	L	R	Pee	Poop
	L	R	Pee	Poop
	L	R	Pee	Poop
	L	R	Pee	Poop
	L	R	Pee	Poop

Breastfeeding my baby is better for the *environment.*

Your breastmilk is a valuable renewable natural resource that is the most ecologically sound food source available. It is produced, (by you) and delivered to the consumer, (your sweet baby) without using other resources, and it creates no pollution. In contrast, artificial baby milk production pollutes our land, air, and water and uses up natural resources.

_____

_____

_____

_____

_____

_____

_____

_____

_____

_____

_____

_____

Time	Minutes on breast		Diaper Changes	
	L	R	Pee	Poop
	L	R	Pee	Poop
	L	R	Pee	Poop
	L	R	Pee	Poop
	L	R	Pee	Poop
	L	R	Pee	Poop
	L	R	Pee	Poop
	L	R	Pee	Poop
	L	R	Pee	Poop
	L	R	Pee	Poop
	L	R	Pee	Poop
	L	R	Pee	Poop

DAY 20

Breastfeeding gives my baby the perfect vitamin and mineral *balance*.

As your baby changes, so will your milk to accommodate your baby's growth. Formula however, can be administered in the wrong amounts and ratios (sleep-deprived parents can measure wrong) and the nutrition in formula is not individually tailored for your baby.

Time	Minutes on breast		Diaper Changes	
	L	R	Pee	Poop
	L	R	Pee	Poop
	L	R	Pee	Poop
	L	R	Pee	Poop
	L	R	Pee	Poop
	L	R	Pee	Poop
	L	R	Pee	Poop
	L	R	Pee	Poop
	L	R	Pee	Poop
	L	R	Pee	Poop
	L	R	Pee	Poop
	L	R	Pee	Poop

I am *preventing* tooth-decay and "baby bottle mouth" by breastfeeding.

Researchers have found that children that were breastfed for more than 40 days were less likely to develop cavities than those who were breastfed for a shorter time. Because of that, the researchers suggest that breastmilk may contain antibodies that inhibit the bacteria that causes tooth decay.

Time	Minutes on breast		Diaper Changes	
	L	**R**	Pee	Poop
	L	**R**	Pee	Poop
	L	**R**	Pee	Poop
	L	**R**	Pee	Poop
	L	**R**	Pee	Poop
	L	**R**	Pee	Poop
	L	**R**	Pee	Poop
	L	**R**	Pee	Poop
	L	**R**	Pee	Poop
	L	**R**	Pee	Poop
	L	**R**	Pee	Poop
	L	**R**	Pee	Poop

DAY 22

Spit-up and baby poop won't stain my *baby's* clothes.

Now you can donate or sell your baby's adorable clothes when they get too small because they aren't permanently stained with formula!

_____

_____

_____

_____

_____

_____

_____

_____

_____

_____

_____

_____

_____

Time	Minutes on breast		Diaper Changes	
	L	R	Pee	Poop
	L	R	Pee	Poop
	L	R	Pee	Poop
	L	R	Pee	Poop
	L	R	Pee	Poop
	L	R	Pee	Poop
	L	R	Pee	Poop
	L	R	Pee	Poop
	L	R	Pee	Poop
	L	R	Pee	Poop
	L	R	Pee	Poop
	L	R	Pee	Poop

DAY 23

Breastfeeding helps to keep my *diet* healthy.

Research has shown that moms who breastfed tend to eat healthier and are more conscious of what they put into their bodies. This creates good habits for their children later on.

Time	Minutes on breast		Diaper Changes	
	L	**R**	Pee	Poop
	L	**R**	Pee	Poop
	L	**R**	Pee	Poop
	L	**R**	Pee	Poop
	L	**R**	Pee	Poop
	L	**R**	Pee	Poop
	L	**R**	Pee	Poop
	L	**R**	Pee	Poop
	L	**R**	Pee	Poop
	L	**R**	Pee	Poop
	L	**R**	Pee	Poop
	L	**R**	Pee	Poop

Breastfeeding my baby will give him/her better *teeth* in the future.

Breastfed babies have better jaw alignment and are less likely to need orthodontic work as they get older. A study of 10,000 children found that those who were breastfed for a year or more were 40 percent less likely to require orthodontic treatment. The sucking action used to breastfeed involves complex motions of the facial muscles and tongue. This improves the development of facial muscles and the shape of the palate.

Time	Minutes on breast		Diaper Changes	
	L	**R**	Pee	Poop
	L	**R**	Pee	Poop
	L	**R**	Pee	Poop
	L	**R**	Pee	Poop
	L	**R**	Pee	Poop
	L	**R**	Pee	Poop
	L	**R**	Pee	Poop
	L	**R**	Pee	Poop
	L	**R**	Pee	Poop
	L	**R**	Pee	Poop
	L	**R**	Pee	Poop
	L	**R**	Pee	Poop

51

DAY 25

Unlike formula, my breastmilk will

never run out!

Did you know that until you wean, milk is being produced at all times, so the breast is never empty. Research has shown that babies do not take all the milk available from the breast - the amount that baby drinks depends upon his appetite.

_____

_____

_____

_____

_____

_____

_____

_____

_____

_____

_____

_____

Time	Minutes on breast		Diaper Changes	
	L	**R**	Pee	Poop
	L	**R**	Pee	Poop
	L	**R**	Pee	Poop
	L	**R**	Pee	Poop
	L	**R**	Pee	Poop
	L	**R**	Pee	Poop
	L	**R**	Pee	Poop
	L	**R**	Pee	Poop
	L	**R**	Pee	Poop
	L	**R**	Pee	Poop
	L	**R**	Pee	Poop
	L	**R**	Pee	Poop

Breastfeeding is *more* convenient!

Your diaper bag will be weighted down with diapers, extra clothes, creams, toys, wipes, etc. But you won't need to carry bottles, formula or water!

_____

_____

_____

_____

_____

_____

_____

_____

_____

_____

_____

_____

_____

_____

_____

_____

Time	Minutes on breast		Diaper Changes	
	L	**R**	Pee	Poop
	L	**R**	Pee	Poop
	L	**R**	Pee	Poop
	L	**R**	Pee	Poop
	L	**R**	Pee	Poop
	L	**R**	Pee	Poop
	L	**R**	Pee	Poop
	L	**R**	Pee	Poop
	L	**R**	Pee	Poop
	L	**R**	Pee	Poop
	L	**R**	Pee	Poop
	L	**R**	Pee	Poop

DAY 27

Breastfeeding my baby *prevents* iron deficiency.

A recent study published by the International Breastfeeding Journal proved that babies who are exclusively breastfed are getting sufficient amounts of iron in their diet, even when the mother is iron deficient.

Time	Minutes on breast		Diaper Changes	
	L	R	Pee	Poop
	L	R	Pee	Poop
	L	R	Pee	Poop
	L	R	Pee	Poop
	L	R	Pee	Poop
	L	R	Pee	Poop
	L	R	Pee	Poop
	L	R	Pcc	Poop
	L	R	Pee	Poop
	L	R	Pee	Poop
	L	R	Pee	Poop
	L	R	Pee	Poop

DAY 28

Breastfeeding my baby is *easier* than the alternative.

Have you seen how many parts some bottles have these days? That is a lot of additional washing! While it may take time and effort to learn how to breastfeed, breastfeeding becomes easier with experience. A breastfed baby's food requires no preparation. Unlike formula, breastmilk from the source is always at the perfect temperature and doesn't spoil. As an additional bonus, the containers are completely portable and they double as comfortably soft pillows for your baby!

Time	Minutes on breast		Diaper Changes	
	L	R	Pee	Poop
	L	R	Pee	Poop
	L	R	Pee	Poop
	L	R	Pee	Poop
	L	R	Pee	Poop
	L	R	Pee	Poop
	L	R	Pee	Poop
	L	R	Pee	Poop
	L	R	Pee	Poop
	L	R	Pee	Poop
	L	R	Pee	Poop
	L	R	Pee	Poop

59

Breastfeeding my baby is *safer!*

Breastmilk is safe, clean, fresh, available, and the most nutritious option for the lowest cost. Formula is a manufactured food containing chemicals, flavorings, vitamins and proteins. The complex processes required to convert these ingredients into food that is digestible by an infant makes formula vulnerable to contamination by bacteria, chemicals, and foreign substances. Between 1982 and 1994, there were twenty-two different recalls of infant formula in the U.S. because of health and safety problems. Seven of these recalls were classified "Class I" - potentially life threatening.

Time	Minutes on breast		Diaper Changes	
	L	R	Pee	Poop
	L	R	Pee	Poop
	L	R	Pee	Poop
	L	R	Pee	Poop
	L	R	Pee	Poop
	L	R	Pee	Poop
	L	R	Pee	Poop
	L	R	Pee	Poop
	L	R	Pee	Poop
	L	R	Pee	Poop
	L	R	Pee	Poop
	L	R	Pee	Poop

61

DAY 30   • *You did it!* •

My baby is *smarter, healthier* and *happier!*

Children who were breastfed have I.Q. scores averaging seven to ten points higher than formula-fed infants. Studies have shown that children who are breastfed get higher grades in school, even after other influences on school performance are taken into account. The intellectual advantage gained from breastfeeding is greater the longer the baby is breastfed. Although intellectual differences between breastfed and formula-fed children used to be attributed to the increased holding and interaction associated with breastfeeding and to the fact that mothers who breastfed were better educated and/or more child-centered, new evidence shows that there are nutrients in breastmilk that enhance brain growth.

62

Time	Minutes on breast		Diaper Changes	
	L	**R**	Pee	Poop
	L	**R**	Pee	Poop
	L	**R**	Pee	Poop
	L	**R**	Pee	Poop
	L	**R**	Pee	Poop
	L	**R**	Pee	Poop
	L	**R**	Pee	Poop
	L	**R**	Pee	Poop
	L	**R**	Pee	Poop
	L	**R**	Pee	Poop
	L	**R**	Pee	Poop
	L	**R**	Pee	Poop

63

Made in the USA
Las Vegas, NV
11 February 2022

43760402R00044